The Enneagram Journey:

Finding The Road Back to the Spirituality Within You - The
Made Easy Guide to the 9 Sacred Personality Types: For Healthy
Relationships in Couples

Sarah Howard & Christian Hope

Table of Contents

Introduction to The Enneagram

Most of us go through life trying to cope with our own struggles, challenges, and demands unaware of the fact that there's a difference between the real self and the ego self of your personality dealing with everyday life. "Being yourself" is easier said than done in our society because we are often embroiled in mass consciousness and the status quo, leaving little room for authentic self-expression and self-understanding. Enter: the Enneagram. It's a tool designed to help you simplify and increase your self-knowledge and transcend your present level of human consciousness in the process.

In a world of illusions, where everyone wears a mask daily, those who have become tired of masquerades are thirsty for truth and authentic self-expression. This is not something new; for centuries now the quest has been going on. There have always been those who have been searching for the real knowledge of who they are since Socrates' time and further back. In our society, however, something is changing.

Humanity is making a momentous leap in consciousness by experiencing the need to develop higher, better, more detailed thinking and behaviours to cope with as our lives become more complex. However, what most of us are discovering is that this approach doesn't work too well.

The best way to thrive as the world continues to make a global shift is not to look for more complicated coping mechanisms to tackle the new emerging world, but rather to simplify the way we relate and partner with life. In other words, we realize that seeking simple solutions to our complex problems is the best option. We're learning to prioritize and appreciate this quest for truth, and we've become curious to find out if there's more to us than we've grown up to believe about ourselves.

Have you reached a point in your life where you need to find out who you've grown like, yet you don't know where to start? Sometimes it can be difficult to understand your own behaviour and actions, or why you react in certain situations as you do. It's a very sobering moment when one day you wake up to realizing you don't even know who you're deep within. The path to the inner world is full of great mystery and can often intimidate us, especially when for decades we have been locked out of our own truth. This is where tools and proven systems are becoming useful.

The Enneagram is an ancient system and tool created to help those of us who care to uncover the layers of mass consciousness so that we can dive to discover our true selves. And this book is designed to help make the journey of self-discovery and this ancient tool simpler, easier to understand and faster to use.

Chapter 1: Origins

The term Enneagram is of Greek origin. Ennea is Greek's number nine, and gram is a drawing. We'd interpret it as a nine-point drawing translated into ordinary English.

In section one of this book, we'll explore in great detail what this drawing looks like and what it means. The critical thing to realize for now is that we're not talking about some new age method to help you cope with life's increasing stresses. There's more to it than meets the eye.

At first, it may seem another one of those entertaining yet juvenile personality tests that have no concrete basis for assuring personal transformation, but if you read through the context of this material and apply proper understanding to it, you will reap the benefits of the contained power.

Some current teachers of this material believe that it's possible to trace variations of the Enneagram symbol to the sacred geometry of Pythagorean mathematicians and mystical mathematicians. While there's a lot of controversy over this theory and who actually originated it, the fact is that it works and is used both in the business world and for spiritual growth. While the Enneagram symbol itself has its roots in ancient times, many individuals have developed the actual system that we use not too long ago today in different ways.

George Gurdijieff, a Russian mystic and teacher is one of those individuals who is credited with the modern reintroduction of the Enneagram symbol. He was a founder of an influential school specialized in' inner work' and his primary way of teaching and using the symbol was through a series of sacred dances or what he called' movements.' He believed in giving his students a direct sense of the meaning of the symbol and the process it represents, but what he did not do was include the ennea-type system as we know it today. We will have to introduce Oscar Ichazo into the story for us to understand who was behind thee system as we know it today.

Oscar Ichazo is credited as the primary individual behind the contemporary Enneagram system. He was a Bolivian man who moved to Peru and later to Buenos Aries in Argentina to study' inner work.' This led to further traveling and searching for wisdom in Asia where he gathered more knowledge across different wisdom traditions that helped him create a systematic way of understanding and applying everything he had learned in his travels. Ichazo combined Taoism, Buddhism, ancient Greek philosophy, Islam, Christianity, and mystical Judaism teachings to form his own school of thought using the ancient Enneagram symbol. Thus from the 1960s, when he began his schooling in Chile, the personality-based Enneagram was offered as a system to help with self-realization and transformation.

The Arica school in Chile, where he taught in the 1960s and early 1970s, was where he first introduced his system of 108 Enneagrams (or Ennneagons, in his terminology). Broadly, these are known as the Passion Enneagram, the Enneagram of the Virtues, the Fixations Enneagram, and the Holy Ideas Enneagram.

During this time in Chile, an American group interested in his work came to South America to study his methods and to experience them firsthand. One of the group's participants was remarkable American psychologist Claudio Naranjo, who recreated his updated version of the personality system of the Enneagram. Although Ichazo and Naranjo began as a teacher and student, each of them went their own way teaching different theories of this Enneagram system and seeing different schools of thought continue to emerge on the subject, don't be surprised to find that some ideas don't always align. Yet, the fundamental goal is not to enter into a debate about who is right or wrong. We are here to develop a healthy understanding of our human psyche. This tool has proven to be very useful to those who practice it and will help you to understand the people around you and yourself better.

Why this matters to you

Understanding why you're acting as you're doing and finding a healthy way to bring out the hidden powers, talents, and aspects of you that would otherwise remain dormant can increase your personal happiness and those of your loved ones. The more you understand why people act as they do, the less likely you're to take things, get discarded or even misunderstand them. There's a greater need for compassion, understanding, and empathy now that we've become more connected than ever as a global community. At work, on social media, at meetings in public, and at home. It helps when human behavior is not such a mystery to you because you can evaluate any given situation and respond rather than react when you have a bearing on the main underlying motives that drive human consciousness.

The bottom line is this.

Anything we can do to know more about ourselves and become better humans is worth diving into and investing a little effort. It takes an open mind and heart, but if you're willing to soak in some new healthy perspectives, I promise to give you insights that can help you.

What This Book Is About

Simply put, this book will answer the big question - Why are you doing what you're doing? It reveals the underlying motives behind each of us, and it will help you to gain clarity on the patterns that do not serve you so that you can improve them as well as shine a light on the positive features that you need to take advantage of.

You will finally discover the real you and become empowered enough to discern the difference between the mask that you wear as a protection. Not only will you learn more about yourself, but with fresh new eyes, you will also begin to see the world understanding why people think, feel, behave and act as they do. This will allow you to detect those that are most compatible with these relationships and to nurture them more. I actually have a chapter that helps you cultivate healthy relationships of love.

I commend you for making this choice to improve yourself and make your fellow human beings better understand. The changes and practices that you integrate as you absorb each chapter will affect your personal success and happiness.

The book is divided into four sections. In section one, we return to the basics so that before integrating this into your life and relationships, you can form a solid foundation. We will dive into the details of the types of Enneagram in section two. In section three, we'll explore more of who you're as well as the Ennea-types subtypes and finally, we'll walk you through integrating this into the most critical areas of your life. You will also have the opportunity to perform an Enneagram test to find out which type and subtype resonates most with you. Now, remember, as is your life, the Enneagram system is a work in progress. Be easy with yourself as you go through this process and try not to get too rigid trying to fit into a particular type or subtype.

The Dark Side of Personality Tests

A woman performed well in her job leading a small team in a major real estate agency until she took one of the most popular personality tests. Her colleagues did not trust her the same way after receiving the results of the personality test. They felt that she didn't have the right personality to be in that position.

In sharing her frustration with me, she said: "Something goes wrong after that day, or I make a mistake that I have this unshakeable feeling that it's because I'm this type of personality and I should be looking for a job that's better suited to that type of personality." This is a real and common problem that many people report once they fall into the downside of relying on shallow personality tests.

The mistake here is fundamental. When we apply rigid labels to ourselves and others that limit the ability to do things outside the test results, it may be like being locked in a small box. I want you to avoid the wrong thinking as we jump into the Enneagram system's basics. You must understand a very simple fact to be able to use this tool effectively.

You're a dynamic, ever-evolving human being. Your experiences, environment, and mindset are changing, and so is your type of personality. This system of nine points is not intended to box you into one category. All nine points are interconnected, and in several types, you can find aspects of you. This is a good thing.

It's possible to be able to find out more about who you truly are and can be done without necessarily fitting into one rigid category. Let's get started.

Section I: Understanding The Basics & Background of The System

Chapter 02: The Theory of Enneagram

If we want a better understanding of the Enneagram and how it's meant to help us lead better lives, we must first consider the primary purpose of Ichazo's work. In reality, every person is perfect, fearless and in loving unity with the entire cosmos; there's no conflict within the person between head, heart, and stomach or between the person and others.

"Then something happens: the ego begins to develop, karma accumulates, there's a transition from subjectivity to objectivity; man falls from essence to personality"

It's about enlightening you and prompting you to wake up to a better understanding of your soul and others ' structure. There's a real self and a day-to-day self that forms the individual you know to be together. Usually we operate our entire life from the ordinary self (also known as the ego-self) that we become alienated from that deep true self and that's where all the inner restlessness, confusion and identity crisis emerges from.

Ichazo developed his transformative teachings and methodologies to help us reconcile these two aspects of ourselves and bring back the harmony and wholeness that is ours. The theory is inspired by the Western mystical and philosophical tradition of nine divine forms as discussed by Plato (platonic solids) and then developed in his work-The Enneads-by the Neo-Platonic philosopher Plotinus in the third century.

These are clearly far from new ideas, but what we can conclude is that no one has effectively consolidated all these different schools of thought into a coherent work. His teaching is based on the fact that, as long as an individual remains in pure essence, they are in complete harmony with life and possess the higher essential qualities also known as the Holy Ideas.

Each Holy Idea has a corresponding virtue. As an individual loses awareness and presence, they fall away from that pure Essence and enter the realm of personality where both the Holy Ideas and the Virtues are distorted into ego-fixation and passion, respectively.

Holy Ideas, Virtues, Ego-fixations, and Passions

According to Ichazo's theory, the loss of self-awareness leads to spiritual contraction, which gives way to ego states. In our thoughts, feelings, and actions, we become distorted and disable the connection with the Divine. He's not saying that we shouldn't have passions and ego-fixations, but pointing out that these are lower untamed aspects of ourselves that are actually part of something bigger and better if we're only learning to use them effectively. It becomes our quest to restore that balance and truth in our lives once we recognize that they are distorted versions of pure essence. This is the primary purpose underlying the Enneagram of personality.

The goal is not just to take a test; it's what happens to you once you take the first step of self-analysis through the test.

14

Chapter 03: Understanding The Modern Day Enneagram

Now that you have context about the purpose and origin of both the ancient Enneagram symbol and the concept behind it, It's time to turn our attention from the basic history to the actual system so that you can begin to see the value it can bring to your life's development.

When you try to understand and study human behavior, there are different approaches that you can use. Most of them involve the diagnosis of pathological behaviors, and while this is important, it's not a very holistic approach and doesn't consider human behavior in its entirety.

What the Enneagram intends to do is offer a more holistic roadmap and a more precise language to help you understand and express what you're discovering about yourself and others. In order to remain relevant, the detailed typing system needed to grow and factor in the psychological discoveries we have made in the modern world.

It's our job to remember that the purpose of this tool is not to label and categorize others or ourselves into certain fixed states. Instead, it's about opening yourself up to recognize the main behavioral patterns that people tend to fall into, understanding that each individual can exhibit any of these personality traits more dominantly than the other traits depending on their present state of being, environment, and how self-aware they are.

In the interview where Claudio Naranjo explained his role in the tool's creation.

He goes on to say that what Ichazo had was a fundamental map that he then helped to develop to a more advanced level

To better understand the Enneagram tool, we need to consider how the mind works. The mind wants to be strategic about managing and navigating life so that you can survive in the best way. The Enneagram's nine-pointed system is said to be the nine distinct and unique qualities that all human beings possess as special characteristics to help an individual navigate life (including trauma).

Your type of Enneagram is the navigation tool that always secretly influences your behaviour, perceptions, and reactions in ways that you may not always predict. The more you can understand the type of your Enneagram, the more insight you will have about yourself and your usual thinking patterns, because you will recognize that there's one primary way you can perceive and react to things that demonstrate your dominant Enneagram personality. This will enable you to make an informed decision as to whether or not you want to activate other characters that you feel are better suited to the type of person you aspire to be.

It will also help you to better discern between the real self and the self in you. It's a subtle yet complex system, but you don't have to be overwhelmed or confused. As we hit this book's core and uncover this nine-pointed system, take a moment to pause between the description of the type and see which ones are resonating with you. Towards the end of the book, we're going to do a simple Enneagram test to help you figure out where you're standing and which type is your personality most dominant. But let's explore in more detail each numbered point and the Enneagram structure for now.

Chapter 04: Introduction To The Different Enneagram Types

Based on the personality system's Enneagram teachings, we know there are nine points. Each of them has a unique name of type.

1. *The Perfectionist also called the Reformer.*
2. *The Giver also called the Helper.*
3. *The Achiever also called the Performer.*
4. *The Romantic also called the Individualist.*
5. *The Observer also called the Investigator.*
6. *The Loyalist also called the Doubter.*
7. *The Enthusiast also called the Dreamer.*
8. *The Challenger also called the Leader.*
9. *The Peacemaker also called the Diplomat.*

However, it's worth mentioning that the system contains more than just these nine types. There are also centers and wings that play a major role in interpreting and understanding your results when taking the test.

Centers:

Centers further arrange the nine points into three groups. On the diagram they form a triad. Classifying the numbered points as the Instinctive Center for Type 1, 8 and 9; the Feeling Center for Type 2, 3 and 4; and finally the Thinking Center for Personality Type 5, 6 and 7.

The Wings:

The wings are what help us to recognize the fact that we are all connected irrespective of type and also that we are not stuck exclusively and rigidly to a numbered point. As a matter of fact, unless we embrace and develop "our wings," it will still be hard to reach our full potential in life.

We dive more into the centers and wings in the next chapter, where you can even get a visual sense of the Enneagram to help you better connect with the system.

As you can see, there are added layers of complexities that can be very intriguing to an individual who is interested. As complicated as this system may seem, it's very dynamic and simple as soon as you understand and connect to the diagram structure itself, because it will give your mind a working mental image from which to grasp more about your natural proclivities.

When you try to find out more about yourself, others and why you're acting as you do, the Internet has a lot of solutions to choose from. Unfortunately, most of them don't have the merit to give you a response that can transform your life. However, the Enneagram personality tool is one of the few globally recognized systems that not only helps you to learn more about your personality, but also expands your awareness to show you how to tap into realms that go far beyond superficial trends. Best of all, it gives you insights into how your personality type will behave when you're exposed to unhealthy, stressful situations and how good things can be when you're on the healthy path of personality development.

Chapter 05: Structure of The Diagram

The structure of the conventional Enneagram diagram is designed to help you connect visually, mentally and emotionally with the tool. I bet you're wondering why the system is numerically numbered 1-9 before we start dissecting it. I was also curious about that. Does a higher numerical ranking mean that there's more value in one personality type compared to another?

Absolutely not! There's no value difference between the larger number and the smaller number. So just because someone is an eight doesn't mean they're better than a three.

I firmly believe no one is better or worse than the other. With different attributes that can be expressed in healthy or unhealthy ways, each character is unique. Certainly, you'll find some people who want a specific number because it's better to be that type of personality according to society, but I just don't agree with that notion. I think that if underdeveloped, any symbol can become a handicap. The key is to nurture the healthy aspects that most resonate with whichever you type. Don't get so upset about what the best personality is "people say." The best character for you is to be authentically yourself and appear as the highest version you can be.

Starting from the outside layers and working your way in is the fastest way to understand the diagram. Imagine a circle drawing. Then inside the circle a triangle and let it touch all three corners. Mark the three points of the triangle 9, 3 and 6 in clockwise position with 9 sitting at the top of the circle.

All you have to do now is make six points equidistant from the circumference of the circle and specify the remaining numbers 1,2,4,5,7 and 8 to fill the gaps. Be sure to do it in a clockwise motion and symmetrically. Each of these numbers is one of the top nine types of personality. If you do this activity by hand, you will begin to notice that internal lines can connect the nine points in some way and that points 3, 6 and 9 actually form an equilateral triangle. You can connect the remaining six points as shown in the diagram below. The importance of these inner lines leads us to another vital lesson when it comes to an understanding of the Enneagram tool.

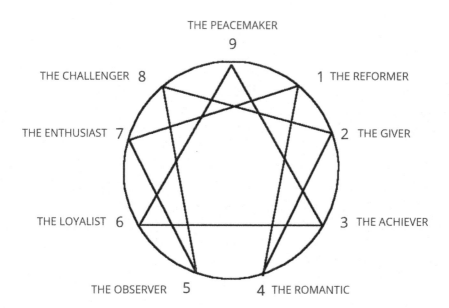

The tool is used to help a person identify their most dominant type within the nine-point system at a fundamental level. There's more to it, though, than those who want to dive deeper. Between the nine points there's also interconnection. So while you may find that your basic personality is a 2, discovering a little more of yourself in all nine types is not uncommon. This is where the Centers and Wings come into play.

All Enneagram teachers and authors agree that we are all born with a specific dominant type of personality that emerges in childhood to help us adapt to our environment.

As infants, we don't really have a developed sense of ourselves. The ego hasn't yet been activated and just spend some time in a park if you're unclear about this. Notice how the small child has no sense of identity in a pram. They can hardly tell the difference between their fingers and their toes or whether or not a doll belongs to them. Then look at the infants who are beginning to become more self-conscious. They can identify their parents and siblings, but they still have no sense of themselves. Then we observe five-year-olds, chasing a ball around. The ball owner knows that it belongs to her, and if you grab it from her, she would probably cry, but the self is still very fluid. Once they reach the age of seven and older, the self is well defined, and it's all about taking ownership and determining "me" and "mine." We developed a sense of self in order to help us fit into this world and survive, depending on our environment, what our caregivers taught us, how they treated us and what we were exposed to.

Therefore, we may generalize that our formative years and everything we have been exposed to help shape our personalities. We learned to rely more heavily on the type of personality that would enable us in the world around us to survive and feel safe. Some of what we ended up choosing may be wonderful, but maybe some aspects are not at all healthy yet we still appear as that person in the world. In addition, we may have neglected to develop and leverage the influences of the connected qualities and special capabilities that we may possess. That's why it can be worthwhile to get to know what center you belong to and what wings you have. Let's discuss further the role of the three centers and the wings before jumping into each of the next section's nine points.

Centers:

As mentioned above, Centers are segmented into a triad. These are intelligence centers that will fall into each of the numbered points. Each center will have three types of personality. The triad consists of the center of thought, the center of feeling, and the center of gut.

Also known as the centers of head, heart, and gut. These centers are deliberately designed and designated for the specific areas on the diagram. Centers are usually differentiated from one another based on how the person usually interprets life and others.

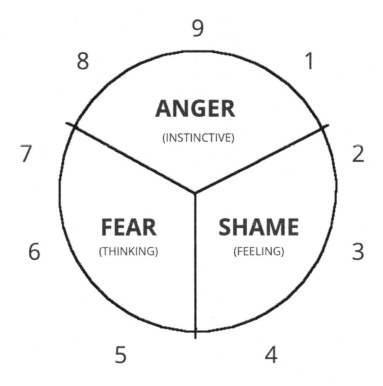

Thinking Center:

Head types are usually too stuck in their heads. They tend to pull out of relationships. The head center is a cognitive center and the people in this triad love thinking, analyzing, and cautiously approaching things. Picture you've been at a party for a moment. If you're part of the center of thought, then your natural tendency and preference would be at or near the door so that you can have a better view and just observe others.

Some authors like to refer to them as mental-based types. Their dominant emotion to keep in check is Fear.

The Feeling Center:

The types of heart are usually people engaging in relationships and continually looking for others. They are very concerned with other people's feelings and interactions. Go back to the scene of the party. Instead of standing by the door this time to see who's present and what's happening around you, you'd be the first to mingle, introduce yourself to people, and try to connect with as many people as possible.

Some people will refer to these types as feeling-based. Their dominant emotion is Shame.

The Instinctive Center:

The types of gut are instinctual. They are very straightforward and have no fear of being confrontational. People tend to act first in this triad and then think and feel later. If we take the last example of this party, you would know if this triad would fit your perfect approach from the moment you entered the room. Are you, in your interaction with others, bold, loud, hearty and jovial? Maybe you're coming off too hard that others often find offensive or intimidating. And if your type of person is not shy when it comes to offering constructive criticism even if it's to the party's host, then I would say this is your center.

Some authors will refer to these types as types based on the body. Anger is the dominant emotion to keep in check here.

According to the Enneagram Institute, each type is the result of a specific relationship with a cluster of issues that characterize that center. Most simply, these issues are about a powerful, mostly unconscious, emotional response to the loss of self-contact.

In other words, you have a particular unconscious emotional response that often surfaces as a result of the loss of contact between the little self of everyday life and the true self. The three centers that have been grouped into Thinking, Instinctive and Feeling centers have as their dominant emotions Fear, Anger and Shame respectively.

So if you take the Enneagram test and discover that you're a type 6 and after a little reflection you realize that fear is one of the greatest paralyzers that holds you back from greatness, then you have just confirmed that you're dominant in that. So when you're improving your life and working hard to manifest a life you love, it's important to keep a close watch on fear because that would be your biggest saboter.

Each intelligence center has certain liabilities and assets that are included in it that will possess the assigned types of personality that come under that group. Type three, for example, falls into the "feeling center," suggesting that their most dominant unconscious emotion is shameful. It also means that they have certain strengths and qualities in relation to "feelings," which is why they fall into that triad.

Just so we're clear, that doesn't mean you're not going to experience other emotions. Think of the group in which you're as having a theme. Whatever your theme is, that will be your most dominant emotion to deal with.

The Wings:

The reason that I believe wings are an important aspect to be included in your interpretation of the results of your Enneagram is that in truth, none of us can be fully summarized by a single personality type.

We are unique and complex people. Always evolving and changing from moment to moment. Our character has to be a combination of different qualities as well. The wings help to integrate this concept into the system.

Although some Enneagram teachers argue that we have only one wing, I am convinced that we need more than one wing. The number 1 is connected to 2 on one side and 9 on the other, even if we judge it from a strictly numerical point of view. The type that is adjacent to the 1 is what we call your wing. Just as you need both wings for a bird or plane to fly, you need wings to soar. These wings compliment your core personality. They connect you to your "closest neighbors," giving you access to various resources and features that can be very useful.

Are both wings equally dominant and do you need to develop each individually?

Yes...and no. It's not an easy question to answer in fact. The Institute of the Enneagram provides some insight into this. "People's observation leads us to conclude that while the two-wing theory applies to some individuals, most people have a dominant one. In the vast majority of people, while the so-called second wing is always operational to some degree, the dominant wing is much more important."

I think the most important thing to remember when it comes to your wings is that you will resonate more with one si. As years go by, this may also change, and you may find yourself switching and displaying more of the less influential wing's qualities. Either way, it's good to be aware of both and figure out which one aligns best with your basic personality and the human being you want to become.

An effective way to approach and understand your wings:

I walked into my favorite frozen yogurt parlor not too long ago to take a break from the hour-long shopping trip I had just finished. Unfortunately, this refreshing break I wasn't the only one I needed. It'd be waiting in line for about 5 minutes before I finally got my turn. Instead of scowling and feeling sorry for myself, I decided to observe with what the people before me were ordering. When I realized how unique we are all, it was a rather exciting experience. Some people wanted no toppings at all but the plain base. Others wanted four different toppings.

An adolescent girl just before me wanted to know if she could get six different toppings! I thought it was a bit too much. I felt quite modest by the time it was my turn when I asked for a frozen yogurt of medium size with just Nutella as the topping! Yes, I'm a junkie for Nutella, what can I tell you?

This is the point of the story...

As we all differ uniquely within our preferences and the relationships with our wings will also vary from individual to individual. The wings are not the frozen yogurt; they are the toppings with which you can choose to flavor your yogurt (type of core personality). We all have access to our two wings, and sometimes one will lean more heavily towards one, or another.

The more you know your preference, the easier it will be to use your wings. Some people absolutely don't like any topping. We'd call them a light wing in this case; some want lots of toppings or too much of one kind. Those we could call strong wings. Others like me want the right amount of toppings, and we can call it balanced double wings. Connecting to your wings can help you to understand the subtleties of your core personality type, regardless of your preference.

As you lean more to one side or the other in your wings, you will expand your perspective and increase your ability to handle tension, creating a greater potential for reframing influencers that no longer serve you. Each core personality type on each side of the nine-point system comes with a connected "close neighbor." In the next section, some of the gifts and challenges that each wing carries will be explored as we unlock the qualities of core personality types. Let's get to it.

SECTION II:

Types of Enneagram Personalities In Detail

Chapter 06: Type One Enneagram of Personality Types

Type One: The Perfectionist, also called the Reformer

Type One's are usually considered. They enjoy a feeling of control and is constantly in need of doing what's best. Some of the core values are integrity and responsibility for this type.

It's critical for those who fall into this first type to be considered a good person, often taking a black and white approach to everything. Something is good or bad

Famous celebrities like Hilary Clinton, Martha Stewart or even world reformers like Nelson Mandela are likely to fall into this type.

Typical qualities are attributed to some. Character traits such as purposeful, principled, self-controlled, integrity-filled and pragmatic.

They may be quite calm and serene, but they are also known to be highly critical of themselves and others. They tend to be very judgmental and uncompromising. Since they fall into the Instinctive Center, rage and anger are common experiences, but they do a good job of suppressing it because they don't really like expressing emotions.

If you're a type one person, you're more likely to be interested in doing the right thing at all times. Common sense is what you believe in, and you're often very responsible for wondering what's wrong with people who don't take life seriously and take responsibility for themselves. You have high standards and you tend to be an idealist doing the best you can to improve the world around you, hence the common term "reformer." You're detail-oriented, accurate in your way of communication, and grounded.

How to improve yourself:

The best way to help your personal growth is to practice being less critical of yourself if you resonate most with type one. Learn to release healthy anger, rage, resentment, or anything else.

It will also be a liberating experience to learn to forgive yourself and others for errors, as it will better empower you to deal with the imperfections you're aware of. Also, allow yourself to have fun!

Your Wings

The Nine Wing:

Gifts: Some of the gifts this wing brings to the strict perfectionist include, but are not limited to the following.

- That strong urge you often have to correct or improve people and things are significantly reduced.
- You can have more points of view and be more open and collaborative.
- There is an increased sense of relaxation, confidence and acceptance.

Type Two: The Giver also called the Helper

This type of person is naturally very empathetic, caring and helpful to others, hence the term "helper."

Think of an iconic figure like Diana-Princess of Wales or Mother Teresa and you have a good understanding of this type of personality. If we dared to go too far, we might even assign this numbered point to religious archetypes like Jesus Christ.

Some qualities are attributed to the twos type. Character traits like authenticity, compassion, generosity, possessiveness, and caring.

Because they have such a strong need for love, they can often become pleasant to people.

Type twos have deep-rooted values that focus on their relationships and puts a lot of energy into them, to the extent that they can sometimes neglect their personal needs. Undoubtedly Empaths would be considered to fall into this category. They are grouped as part of the Feeling Center, being a feeling-based type, and this unfortunately leads to the dominant sense of shame.

Often a person in this category will try to mask the shame they're experiencing and that feeling of not being good enough by overcompensating their interactions with others so that people can think of them as good.

If you're a type two personality, then you're more likely to be an emotional sponge that's always experiencing more than others, which makes you really good at supporting and giving. But you may have realized that it's a bit tricky to give yourself or take time to meet your needs. On autopilot, you need to be careful not to absorb emotions, as this will destabilize your sense of being grounded. You're a caring, communicative and naturally generous person, but you have to make sure that it doesn't happen from a place of dependence.

How to improve yourself:

Make self-care and self-love a priority in your life. Train yourself to take care of your own needs. I know saying no and setting boundaries is difficult but you have to start recognizing when to set boundaries for your own mental, emotional, spiritual and physical protection.

Your Wings

The One Wing:

Gifts: Some of the gifts this wing brings to the helpful type of giver include but are not limited to the following.

- You may feel more influenced by being more generous and not just giving. It helps you to realize that you don't have to do everything on your own.

Challenges: Some of the challenges this wing brings to the helpful type of giver include but are not limited to the following.

- As you become more involved with work and less involved with your inner self, you may end up neglecting your needs and becoming a workaholic. Hence the danger of excessive pride as the reason for your work.

Type Three: The Achiever also referred to as the Performer

An achiever, commonly referred to as the performer, is the term given to type three personalities. While some similarities exist between type one and three, a person in this category is driven more by success and the best in life. They wants to be admired and validated.

Type threes are hard-working, diligent, and sometimes even somewhat obsessive, which is excellent because it keeps them going until they achieve their objectives. Being the best is something that really cares about this type of personality, and that's why they often become the top performers in their chosen industry. Individuals such as Muhammad Ali, Will Smith, Tom Cruise, Elon Musk, and Oprah Winfrey would undoubtedly be classified as achievers in our modern world.

The qualities this person possesses can be outstanding, and it can also be quite harmful if they focus on the wrong thing. The desire to be the best at work, look good, demonstrate success and always win can make a Type Three super competitive, tense and may even lead them to step over others just to get ahead.

Certain qualities are attributed to this Type Three such as: being driven, self-confident, image-conscious, adaptable, focused, determined, excellent, energetic and great in leadership and communication. This type of personality loves to look good and is usually a smart and wonderful person to learn from when you want to excel in life as well. They have a lot of energy and enthusiasm for life that many find contagious, and this really helps them as they raise up the ranks in life or become self-made successes.

They too fall into the Thinking Center, meaning that shame is an underlying emotional theme that they have to deal with on an ongoing basis. Because the three are so focused on image and outward success, it's usually difficult for him or her to know how to handle emotions, particularly shame. For type threes, denial is often the preferred option.

Their coping mechanism for shame strives to become what they believe to be the most valuable and successful individual they can possibly be, in the hope that this will dissolve that underlying restlessness and feelings of shame and inadequacy.

If you're a type three personality then productivity, high performance and excellence move the needle for you. You love to be the best and to be recognized for it. Forward momentum, you're naturally motivated and motivated to succeed by others around you. There's no doubt about it, you think differently, you dream bigger than most people, and you're trying to achieve more than most people. Your energy is often contagious, and people usually love to be around you because you fire them up.

How to improve yourself:

Take some time to regularly audit yourself and acquire clarity about what true success and happiness mean to you. Looking inside may be a bit frightening, but this is where your real power lies.

Material success must not be confused with fulfillment and self-worth, and you must draw your power from the real Source of Life, not from the power of the agency. Titles, awards and external validation can not be your true value. And that deep sense of meaning that you long for in your life will not come from accomplishments, which is why taking the time to go inside and find out who you really are will enable you to emerge better and more prosperous in every conceivableway.

Your Wings

The Two Wings:

Gifts: Some of the gifts this wing brings to the achievement type include, but are not limited to, the following: It allows you to appreciate people and the contribution they make in your life.

- You also become more aware of your needs and see the value of prioritizing non-work relationships.

Challenges: Some of the challenges this wing brings to the competitive achievement include but are not limited to the following.

- You may experience much more disappointment and self-criticism if your accomplishments are successful. Pleasant people may take a toll on your actions.

The Four Wing:

Gifts: Some of the gifts this wing brings to the competitive attainder include but are not limited to the following.

- One of the best gifts you will receive from this wing is the realization that self-development and time to understand the inner world has tremendous value.

Type Four: The Romantic also called the Individualist

A type four person is mostly referred to as the individualist, but I also like the term romantic.

This person is super creative, he sees beauty and magnificence in everything and tends to romanticize things. Think of famous people like Oscar Wilde, Michael Jackson, William Shakespeare, or the Persian poet Hafiz, and you now have a better idea of people who would fall into this type.

Character qualities associated with this type of personality include creativity, authenticity, courage, passion, and emotional depth.

However, they can also considered very temperamental, self-absorbed, and dramatic. Type fours have an underlying sense of melancholy because they invariably feel like something is missing.

Fours are long to be understood and treasured for who they really are, but they regularly feel misunderstood and disappointed. Such a person will create an inner mental landscape where he feels more liberating and nourishing as a way to escape from the harsh, cruel world that never "gets them" them or their sensitivities.

It has been said that the majority of fours are artistic or very much artistic as a means of self-expression, but whether this is the case or not, a type four personality will tend to experience a great deal of disappointment and dissatisfaction in the world as they feel different and unique from those who are not like them. And in some idealistic way they will try to find and express wholeness and beauty.

Being the most emotional of all types of personality, they tend to struggle the most with the dominant emotional theme of shame. They are part of the Feeling Center and undoubtedly "feel" deeply, so their discomfort is likely to be more pronounced and easier to spot. However, they try to mask this by focusing on how unique and special they are, even though it may lead to rollercoaster experiences plunging into deep depression and other negative emotions to the other extreme of beauty, joy, fantasy, and inspired creativity.

If you're a type four personality, then you value individualism and self-expression. You love to see someone sharing their feelings authentically, yet you notice that sometimes you can be really warm and welcoming, while at other times you can get people dry and almost cold. You can be ecstatic one day and plunge into depression soon after. Envy and jealousy often rage on you even though you don't even like to admit it to yourself.

How to improve yourself:

That inner critic, often so loud, needs to be tamed and put on silent. Internalizing blame is very unhealthy for you and requires a shift in your perception and how negative emotions and situations are processed.

Learn to openly speak your truth without losing your emotional control. Find a way to balance your emotional rollercoaster so you can stop falling into the pit of despair and depression.

Your Wings

The Two Wings:

Gifts: Some of the gifts this wing brings to the creative, intense individualist type include but are not limited to the following.

- The desire to be successful and look good that comes organically from this wing actually helps you to be real. In short, you're more capable of balancing your inner and outer world.

Challenges:

Some of the challenges this wing brings to the creative, intense individualistic type include, but are not limited to, the following.

- There is a tendency to want to fix others and the outer world instead of yourself.
- You're more likely to be agitated and depressed as the ongoing performance pressure builds throughout your life.

Type Five: The Observer also called the Investigator

The Observer personality, commonly referred to as the Investigator is usually brilliant, highly intellectual, keen on learning on an ongoing basis, and is most comfortable in the realm of thinking. This type of person tends to be very independent, enjoying loneliness. They enjoy gathering information and observing patterns all around them trying to make sense of their world and environment. Individuals such as Albert Einstein, Nikola Tesla, Isaac Newton, and Marie Curie are just a few examples of such people.

Some of the qualities associated with type fives are innovative, self-reliant, isolated, secret, curious, perceptive, scholarly, quiet and reserved. They are intense, intelligent thinkers and take great pleasure in tending to their mind's affairs rather than trying to fit into the world.

As mental-based types, fives will often detach themselves from relationships, and many will consider them to be emotionally inexpressive. But they're not all. Some fives care about family and relationships, but it takes a lot of time to recreate and pursue their passions alone. It's not easy to figure out what's going on under a five's surface level and they have an exaggerated need for privacy.

Type five personality falls into the' Thinking Center ' group making fear one of the dominant negative themes they have to deal with. Fear of inadequacy is one of the great battles that must be overcome when dealing with the outside world because they feel unable to actively handle the outside world. Maybe that's why they tend to be detached and their own feelings from others.

Expert says that fives like to leave the open world because of their unconscious fear and belief that they can better relate to it by going into their minds and using it to penetrate the nature of our society. Unfortunately, that usually doesn't work too well for them and in their fear of being overwhelmed by people or emotions they may find arrogant and dismissive.

If you're a type five, then you're likely to value knowledge and continuing education a lot, especially in the topics you're interested in. Some people think you're too intellectual and you may be quite literal at times, but you don't really care.

Small talk and gossip are annoying you and you prefer isolation. You tend to get stuck in your head and prefer to hang out with people who give you plenty of room to think about things. You like to be thorough in everything you do, and you enjoy deep, meaningful conversations very much. In fact, you can talk about it in great technical details for a very long time when you're passionate about something. Reconnecting with your body and heart's sensations and energy is a task even though you know it's good for you and, above all, personal freedom and autonomy bring you great pleasure.

How to improve yourself:

Start by increasing the amount of time you spend reconnecting with your body and emotions. Your ability to gain access to your energy and higher perceptions of the spirit will only strengthen you.

Create for yourself a safe environment where you can regularly embark on this quest so that you can combine your intellectual strength with your spiritual strength.

Put a little more effort into the relationships you care about.

Let your loved ones know you care about them and be more expressive of your feelings, even if you feel a little uncomfortable about them. Let yourself feel emotions like happiness, being in love, gratitude, affection, etc. This will open a channel for others to pour the same into your life and help you deal with the feelings of loneliness and inadequacy that sometimes resurface.

Your Wings

The Two Wings:

Gifts: Some of the gifts this wing brings to the quiet expert type include but are not limited to the following.

- You will have the unusual ability to connect your river for a type five personality.

Type Six: The Doubter also referred to as the Loyal Skeptic

A type six personality is always alert and conscious of their environment and responsibilities. Knowing the rules and protecting those who are under their care is extremely important to sixes. They are very trustworthy and the people they care about value being there. Unfortunately, between trusting and distrusting others, they tend to feel conflicted. They often bounce with a tendency to doubt themselves and question others between skepticism and certainty.

They are very sober-minded people and take problem-solving rather seriously to the point where it becomes a burden on them. For a six, worry and anxiety are common emotions. In this type, peace of mind is always lacking, and they usually struggle with a profound sense of insecurity. If you want an idea of celebrities that could be classified as type six individuals, think of Ellen DeGeneres, Tom Hanks, and Richard Nixon.

Some of the character qualities associated with type six include trustworthy, responsible, committed, loyal, and trustworthy.

The six also fall into the' Thinking Center ' making fear (which often turns out to be worried and anxious) the more dominant emotions.

Stress levels for a six are always high and worry seems to be a constant companion as their life outlook is often quite negative. They will focus more on the negatives than on the positive ones of any given situation.

If you're a type six, then you tend to pay close attention to people and issues. You're really good at anticipating issues and creating solutions, and in others you tend not to like ambiguity. But you may have realized that you could become very pessimistic, doubtful, and even project on other people some of your fears. Sometimes you like playing the Devil's advocate. As you grow, it becomes more important to overcome the disconnect between the mind and the body, and even if you're cautious (maybe even phobic), you're also showing a lot of courage as you try to move forward even when fear holds on to you.

How to improve yourself:

Find ways to deal with the crippling effects of fear in your life and get better at directly addressing it. Ask an expert or trusted friend for some help and support.

Learn to take things with a light heart.

Reconnect more with your body and feelings and create a safe space to do so in order to relax your mental processes and help in this new experiment. The more comfortable and safe you feel mentally, the faster and more enjoyable the mental-body connection will become.

Your Wings

The Five Wing:

Gifts: Some of the gifts this wing brings to the loyal skeptic type include but are not limited to the following.

- This wing helps you make more reasonable and sound decisions. It also makes you open-minded and able to take multiple perspectives.
- You will also experience a deeper sense of inner trust and self-confidence as an observer and authority on your focused interest. This helps to eradicate the need to seek validation from others.

Challenges:

Some of the challenges this wing brings to the loyal skeptic type include but are not limited to the following.

- This wing may amplify your fears and anxiety or any sense of inadequacy that you may have.
- You may notice a tendency to be too stuck in your head and not aligned enough with your feelings. You begin to see more good and become less inclined to imagine the worst of people and the world at large.
- You may notice a shift inside and outside of how you approach others, how playful, lighthearted and enthusiastic you feel. It's even possible to realize and even laugh at your own fears as you see them.

Challenges:

Some of the challenges this wing brings to the loyal skeptic type include but are not limited to the following.

- This wing will amplify the common tendency to fear and avoid pain at all costs. This may lead you to seek

all sorts of unhealthy distractions or to withdraw even more from life.
- Instead, you may start to avoid confronting issues that require your attention and seek escapism.

Type Seven: The Dreamer also called the Enthusiast

The dreamer is spontaneous, a real pleasure seeker and loves to live life to the maximum.

Having fun is the top priority of this type of personality and they always seek to catch the next exciting adventure just around the corner. Also known as enthusiasts or epicures, seven are mental-based types that are forward-thinking and can't be limited to just one thing. They believe in unlimited opportunities, and it demonstrates their variety of passions and interests. Think about people such as Steve Jobs, Robert Downey Jr., George Clooney, and Elton John. We believe they would definitely fall into this type of personality.

Some of the primary qualities attributed to those in this type of personality include enthusiasm, spontaneity, resourcefulness, adventure, optimistic fun and exciting.

Some seven are extroverts though not all of them are great communicators in general. Unfortunately, being mental-based types, they are part of the' Thinking Center' which makes the dominant emotional theme of fear their greatest hurdle to overcome. And it appears in the form of avoiding pain for a seven.

As a seeker of pleasure, a seven will do anything to prevent pain and sometimes seek distractions that turn into overindulgence. But in order to avoid suffering, they rationalize and justify this downward tendency. Also, as they shift so frequently into the next big thing, sevens tend to be very scattered, making it difficult for them to dive deeply into any single idea, or stay the course in relationships and at work. True devotion is hard for a seven because they are such believers in "the next big thing" that makes it hard to narrow down their vision and concentrate wholeheartedly on one thing.

They are usually known as "big talkers" and prone to addiction and over-stimulation, which can be in the form of substance use, gambling, shopping, adventure seeking. It's easy for you to multi-task and you hate the feeling of constriction.

Everything you do has to be fun because it's who you're. You're definitely a multi-passionate human being, so the commonly preached idea of finding your "one thing" is meaningless to you. You love learning new things and with an optimism that others truly admire approach life.

Yet you don't really care about "saving face" or getting people impressed. You just care to do your own thing while at it and have an epic time. You can bounce back very quickly from negative emotions and situations. But deep down, you've come to realize you can't stand the pain experience and it scares you. Negative states of mind, depression, and suffering are unbearable whether they are your own or others. Introspection is not something you enjoy, and you go through cycles of anxiety and desperation that drive you to seek remedies at any cost.

How to improve yourself:

Create a secure support structure that allows you to cope with your pain, loss, deprivation or any other suffering you have avoided. Learn to embrace your inner world and reconnect with it.

48

Be more present at the moment and find peace of mind and comfort without using stimulants. It won't be easy, I'm not saying it will be, but you can do it.

With your level of intelligence, resourcefulness, creativity, natural strength and optimism you can gain true freedom and enjoy being the expanding, adventurous human you were meant to be while remaining grounded in your true self.

Your Wings

The Six Wing:

Gifts: Some of the gifts this wing brings to the enthusiast include but are not limited to the following. It creates a sense of seriousness and motivates your desire for unlimited freedom.

Challenges:

Some of the challenges this wing might bring to the enthusiast include, but are not limited to, the following.

- That increased sense of duty might potentially begin to feel like a burden.
- Your underlying fears may appear to be amplified, self-doubt may increase, and you may end up feeling guilty. If your selfish desires combine with a need for immediate satisfaction, then in the name of pleasure and gain you might run the risk of going too far. Even if it means making the most of others to get what you want.
- You may become more self-absorbed and look down on others and treat them with a sense of superiority.

49

Type Eight: The Challenger also called the Leader

The best statement to summarize this type of personality is *"I am a master of my fate. I am the captain of my soul."* Indeed, this type of personality believes in taking full control of their lives and being perceived as the powerful, active leader and protector. Justice, fairness, and independence for type eight are of great value. They will fight back with vengeance if wrong.

Eights are body-based types that give them strong physical appetites and strong instincts. They are bold, they are active in making decisions, they love to be independent and they are very intense people. A person typed as an eight generally desires a great life, and They is ready to go out and fight for that desire. In our modern world, individuals such as Donald Trump embody this type.

Some of the qualities attributed to type eights include self-confidence, courage, willingness, determination, power, courage, generosity, and domination.

Eights can sometimes be difficult to handle, especially if their personalities have been developed in unhealthy ways. They are predisposed to make their emotional theme anger in the 'Instinctive Center'. Type Eights really know how to get angry. Whenever they don't get their own way, or things go wrong, they're very quick to anger, and that anger can quickly turn into rage and physical violence if it remains unchecked.

They produce a lot of energy to meet challenges with the right mental and physical attitude. A feeling of weakness is the one thing an eight can't stand. Vulnerability (based on how it's defined by society) is also something that a type eight would keep clear of, making it difficult to have a deep and intimate relationship with the type eight.

They still need to feel in control and powerful even in their intimate relationships. Eight are fierce when it comes to protecting their family, friends, and their caregivers. They're going to go to the ends of the earth and do whatever it takes to accomplish the mission.

If you're a type eight personality, you've noticed a tendency to be excessive within you. Some people call you bossy even if you don't get the reason. You see it as being firm, focused, clear, assertive, and leading to victory for others.

Idleness, weakness, shyness are all things that you can not stand in yourself and others, and you prefer when people address you directly and confidently. You may get outraged when provoked, and you tend to be vengeful towards people. But you keep an open mind.

How to improve yourself:

you have a lot of energy. Probably the most energetic of all the nine types, which means that you need to constructively direct that energy. Incorporate some self-control into your life and do not allow your automatic reaction to remain anger and aggression just because it's a comfortable habit.

Redefine your meaning of vulnerability and learn to receive love and affection. Request help from someone you trust or hire an expert if you need some personal assistance and support. It's not a kind of weakness. Don't get caught up in this false belief. Improving yourself is a form of strength and empowers you to become a better leader and protector.

Your Wings

The Seven Wings:

Gifts: Some of the gifts this wing brings to the active controller include but are not limited to the following.

- Tapping into this wing's gifts will calm you down, increase your happiness and help you move more enthusiastically through life. It gives you a light heart and dissolves some of that ruthlessness that often rules your life.
- Instead of being a lone wolf trying to make it all yourself, you'll start to value connecting with other people, exchanging ideas, expressing your thoughts and acting out your fantasies in a more harmonious way.

Type Nine: The Peacemaker also called the Diplomat

A Type Nine is generally known as someone that "goes with the flow" in life. Above all, they value harmony, peace and balance and do whatever they can to avoid conflict and rivalry. Individuals like the Dalai Lama, Queen Elizabeth II, Abraham Lincoln, and Grace Kelly are all great examples of people of this type of personality.

Some of the essential qualities associated with this type of personality include tolerance, robustness, reliability, soundness, calmness, and goodwill.

Nines are body-based types that love to get along with everyone and are pretty awesome to be around. Nines can tolerate a lot and usually approach every situation in an optimistic manner. They like seeing the best in others and have a strong belief that things are always going to work for the best. They believe in a friendly universe and want to have as much as possible an open mind and heart.

They are grouped in the 'Instinctive Center' to watch out for their dominant emotional theme. All this calmness, if left unchecked, can turn into something dark and unhealthy. And it happens mostly in the form of emotions suppressed and denied.

Because of the inherent desire to be a peace-maker in the world, nines generally deny the threatening emotions of anger that arise so frequently. With their instinctual drives and dominant emotions in this area, they are the most out of touch with these baser emotions. Their need to avoid conflict at all costs (including internal conflict) causes their unpleasant hidden feelings to become repressed. A nine is also prone to inaction and procrastination, particularly when They senses unpleasant emotions.

If you're a type nine personality, then you value the profound connection with the world and those you care about. You tend to change in a conservative way and sometimes struggle with a lack of motivation. Being out in nature gives you the most satisfying feeling

People think you're warm, nurturing, reliable and attentive. This self-sacrificing tendency, however, carries some significant disadvantages that you don't like to face up to as it causes discomfort. You may notice that people are beginning to take you for granted or undervalue everything you're doing for them, and it can be very discouraging. You have a tendency to "forget yourself" as you easily merge with others that make it really hard for you to create personal boundaries.

How to improve yourself:

Call yourself to take more risks in life. Create a safe space in your life where you can train yourself to integrate harmony and conflict so you can stop avoiding them all the time.

Pay more attention to your own needs and learn to set clear boundaries. Reconnect with your emotions and embrace conflict or anger discomfort as it appears within you so that you can deal with it boldly. Instead of suppressing the negative emotions that appear. Give yourself time and space to process all your feelings.

With your top priorities, be more structured and strategic. If it's a matter of getting more organized then ask for help or acquire one of the many modern tools to help you better prioritize activities on a daily basis.

Your Wings

The Eight Wing:

Gifts: Some of the gifts this wing brings to the adaptive peacemaker include but are not limited to the following.

- The positive influence this wing has on your core personality as a peacemaker. It will help you build some structure around your life and activities. You will develop a more focused perspective and lead a principle-based life.
- Instead of accepting dysfunction as the standard way of life, you will feel empowered to be more actively involved in changing things that go wrong. You will be more action-oriented, but it will come from a place of purpose and certainty.

Challenges:

Some of the challenges this wing brings to the adaptive peacemaker include but are not limited to the following:

- The increased need to do what is right and make the world perfect may lead to even more procrastination and distraction. The fear of not getting it right may actually become a huge obstacle.
- You may be caught in the trap of doing what you "should do" or what you're expected to do rather than what you really want to do.

Section III: Instincts, Subtypes and variants within the Enneagram of Personality Tool

Chapter 07: Diving Deeper into who you really are

Like animals, we as humans have continued to evolve has physical and conative beings. Our evolution has required us to develop strategies that will allow us to survive and extend our species' life on this planet. What the Enneagram does, is facilitate a better understanding of the instinctual strategies that we have developed as human beings, and shows us how it affects a person's behaviour in different ways. This is more than just getting to know your personality type; it's about pulling back the curtain of the influences that drive you to act as you do.

There are three basic human instincts that the Enneagram teachers, and out of these three we see a detailed dissection of how these instincts interact and combine with the nine types of personality. These are:

- Instinct for self-preservation.
- Social Instinct.
- Sexual Instinct.

All three instincts are within us and often ruling unconsciously behind our life strategies. While these three are always present, one tends to dominate more, and we tend to prioritize and develop that particular drive while the other tends to be less dominant. And because we don't make improving the least dominant one a priority, it tends to become our blind spot.

Think of these three instincts as you'd be a layered cake. At the top we have our most controlling one, in the middle we have the second one that supports the predominant one, and at the bottom we have the least developed instinct.

Again, even here we find some conflict with some schools stating that they should not be referred to as subtypes, while others teach that they are actually subtypes of the nine-point system. Anyway, we don't care about the label. We're only concerned with how we can better understand who we are and why we're acting as we do. The primary instinct with which we identify in combination with our personality type of Enneagram helps shape our life path and the choices we make.

Since that is our core focus, after a brief understanding of what each instinct entails, we will dive into each of the twenty-seven combinations.

Instinct for self-preservation:

The need to preserve our body and its life force. Keep away from threats. This includes our basic human needs for food, shelter, clothing, warmth, and family relationships.

This instinct is highly focused on physical well-being, safety, material safety, and everyday comfort. Every time our basic needs are threatened by the environment, we can use resource and energy hoarding to preserve what we have as a result of the external threat. We may consider this as the basic primal instinct possessed by all creatures. The drive for survival and self-preservation.

Social Instinct:

This social instinct is also called "the adaptive" instinct.

It's the need to get along with others and form secure social bonds. It's about creating a sense of belonging around you.

Today we see this a lot on social media with memberships and communities emerging where like-minded people (who feel the need to belong) are gathering. It's about focusing energy on working for shared purposes or the greater good.

This instinct is very much about being part of something that resonates with you where you feel secure, heard and valued within that group and community.

Sexual Instinct:

Sexual Instinct is also called "attraction" instinct.

It's the universal need to procreate and pass on our genes to continue. It governs our sexuality, intimacy, and the close friendships we cherish.

This instinct also directs the vitality of the life force within our bodies. It focuses on the intensity and passion contained in experiences and one on one relationship that leads us to search for opportunities that promise strong alliances, synergy, and deep connections.

This instinct is often confined to just sexual intimacy, but it's meant to be so much more. It's definitely about projecting yourself into the environment and experiencing intimate relationships that are pleasurable and extending your DNA, but it can also be about passing on ideas that help you create a legacy that goes far beyond your physical reach.

When we overlay these three human behaviour instincts with everything we've talked about so far, the end result is a combination of twelve. The set of combinations that falls into our most dominant type of personality helps us to connect with the intricacies of our daily behaviour and preferences.

"These instincts relate to the fundamental instinctual intelligence that develops within each of us to ensure our survival as individuals and as a human species.

Recent advances in neuroscience research have confirmed the strong and often invisible intelligence.

Self Preservation Instinct	Social Instinct	Sexual Instinct
The need to preserve our body and its life force. Keeping away from threats. This includes our basic human needs of food, shelter, clothing, warmth and family relations.	The need to get along with others and form secure social bonds. It's about creating a sense of belonging around you.	The universal need to procreate and continue the human race generation after generation. It governs our sexuality, intimacy and the close friendships that we treasure as well as our legacy.
Type 1: The Perfectionist /Reformer	**Type 1: The Perfectionist /Reformer**	**Type 1: The Perfectionist /Reformer**
• Anxiety	• Non-adaptability	• Zealousness or Jealousy
Type 2: The Giver/Helper	**Type 2: The Giver/Helper**	**Type 2: The Giver/Helper**
• Privilege	• Ambition	• Seduction or Aggression
Type 3: The Achiever/Performer	**Type 3: The Achiever/Performer**	**Type 3: The Achiever/Performer**
• Security	• Prestige	• Charisma
Type 4: The Romantic/Individualist	**Type 4: The Romantic/Individualist**	**Type 4: The Romantic/Individualist**
• Fearlessness	• Shame	• Competition
Type 5: The Observer/Investigator	**Type 5: The Observer/Investigator**	**Type 5: The Observer/Investigator**
• Castle	• Symbols	• Confidant
Type 6: The Loyalist/Doubter	**Type 6: The Loyalist/Doubter**	**Type 6: The Loyalist/Doubter**
• Warmth	• Duty	• Warrior
Type 7: The Enthusiast/Dreamer	**Type 7: The Enthusiast/Dreamer**	**Type 7: The Enthusiast/Dreamer**
• Networking	• Sacrifice	• Fascination
Type 8: The Challenger/Leader	**Type 8: The Challenger/Leader**	**Type 8: The Challenger/Leader**
• Survival	• Camaraderie	• Possessiveness
Type 9: The Peacemaker/Diplomat	**Type 9: The Peacemaker/Diplomat**	**Type 9: The Peacemaker/Diplomat**
• Strong Appetite	• Participation	• Fusion

Personality Type One: The Perfectionist also called the Reformer

Self-preservation Instinct:

The basic character drive here will be projected as anxiety.

This is the perfectionist who is constantly concerned and seeking to control everything. Their anxiety causes them to constantly try to anticipate risks, and they like to be prepared for it all. For them, attention to detail is likely an understatement. Usually they are very hard on themselves and take things rather seriously.

This subtype prefers to avoid expressing anger even if they feel it, and when interrupted they will often experience and show great frustration. The type one subtype has a very loud inner critic and tends to amplify their anxiety and worry.

Social Instinct:

The basic character drive here will be projected as Non-adaptability.

Fairness and making things right motivates this subtype. They are systematic thinkers, set high standards for themselves and others, and like being an example of integrity and principled conduct.

They practice a lot of self-control and can be quite friendly while in their own comfort zone. Because they are so linear and see everything in black and white, it can be hard to adapt to a new environment or situation, right or wrong. They can also become very resentful and critical with those who don't fit their right idea.

Sexual Instinct:

The basic character drive here will be projected as zealousness and/or jealousy.

This subtype will be highly charged, passionate and maintain high self-control standards. They have an idealistic view of how things should be and tend to want to reform others and fit them into "what's right."

Rage and anger will be expressed directly by those who fall into this subtype, especially if their efforts to improve others are restricted. They also prioritize their partner's attention and are usually very jealous of their partner or other people who seem to do better.

2. Personality Type Two: The Giver also called the Helper

Self-preservation Instinct:

The basic character drive here will be projected as Privilege.

This type two feels privileged and unique in some way because it invests heavily in creating warm nurturing relationships. They spend a lot of time looking after others and supporting them. As such, there's a tendency to become self-titled and even develop a prideful attitude that requires special privileges and approval as a result of care.

They are "nice" with a highly activated childlike spirit. This type two likes to be looked after but is not too keen on long-term commitments. Fear of rejection is a great deal for this subtype, and they can experience a great deal of hurt and abandonment when their needs are not met.

Social Instinct:

The basic character drive here will be projected as Ambition.

Forming the right alliances and having great allies is essential for this subtype because they want to build their self-esteem through visible achievements and social achievements.

They enjoy taking on leadership roles and standing out from the crowd. They enjoy "being on" and build their influence based on the connections they form as well as their skills.

Those in this subtype do not actively demonstrate a child-like spirit (at least not as much as the other type twos) and tend to have a strategy of giving more than they get. Seeking recognition through ambition is more pronounced in this type of two personalities.

Sexual instinct:

The basic character drive here will be projected as Seduction and/or aggression.

This type two will focus all their energies, abilities and seductive abilities in forming and nurturing powerful and intimate relationships.

This type of person is passionate, resilient, strong-willed and willing. They are very devoted in their personal relationships, and they don't like taking no for an answer.

This type two uses seduction, which can go as far as turning into aggression if pushed into it, to gain the desired attention and recognition.

Although they like to use body language and feeling tones that can be found as seductive, it doesn't necessarily imply sexual desire.

3. The Achiever also called the Performer

Self-preservation Instinct:

The basic character drive here will be projected as Security.

This type three variation is highly focused on accomplishment and creating material success for itself. This type of person avoids being viewed as image-oriented and doesn't openly like to advertise their strengths. But it's still very important to them to be successful and to get recognition for their hard work. Financial success and the creation of a sense of security around them is an enormous priority for this subtype.

They work very hard and like to maintain high standards and a good image of success. This subtype three has an abundance of energy and tends to accomplish a lot.

The real danger for them is that they often lose contact with their authentic self in pursuing all that success and are prone to creating false identities and valuing themselves on the basis of their job role or social status.

Social Instinct:

The basic character drive here will be projected as Pr.

This type three variation is more interested in validating and receiving lots of social endorsement. They crave power, work hard to "know the right people" and focus a lot on gaining powerful leadership positions in government or business.

Prestige, praise, and influence are what this subtype will be after most, and they will generally train themselves to adjust to teams or organizations ' social norms and requirements if it helps them gain influence and power. They are highly competitive and love to be at the center of attention.

This particular subtype will have no problems promoting their ideas and achievements with confidence. Unlike the first type three who prefer not to advertise their achievements and success, this subtype would actually go to the extreme to make known theirs. And to cover up anything that doesn't align with that "perfect image of success."

Sexual Instinct:

The basic character drive here will be projected as Charisma.

Personal power and gender identification as well as all the issues that arise from that mostly drive three variations of this type. They have a lot to do with masculinity and femininity. Having a "movie star" life that means having the perfect outer image is what rocks your world. They are also very enthusiastic and charismatic, making them very likable.

It's very important to be attractive to others as a man or woman. But they also enjoy supporting others in their success and often have that enthusiastic attitude "if you succeed, I succeed."

The biggest challenge for this subtype, despite remaining very competitive, charismatic and powerful on the outside, is that those who fall into their subtype's unhealthy path often quietly struggle with confusing feelings about their sexuality. Tackling such conflicts can be tough as there's so much effort to appear as a powerful performer.

4. The Romantic also called the Individualist.

Self-preservation Instinct:

The basic character drive here will be projected as Fearlessness.

This type four variation will express their emotions less while still being very sensitive and idealistic. In a sense, we could say that the three subtypes are the least dramatic. But that doesn't mean they don't experience those tumultuous emotions, they just want to be seen as someone who doesn't complain.

The truth is that this type of person has just trained themselves to live with pain and suffering. They know how to internalize negative emotions and prefer being tough enough to deal with anything that comes along. Compared to the other subtypes, it makes them less likely to open up and share their feelings with others, but this doesn't mean that they lack empathy. In fact, they are trying very hard to reach out to and support those who are suffering around them.

This subtype is very creative and profoundly anxious to experience an authentic life, even though that sometimes means being a little reckless. They will have no trouble packing up and moving into a completely new environment if their self-preservation trigger makes them feel like an authentic experience is elsewhere.

The biggest challenge for this variation of personality type is the tension often created between the desire to build material security in their lives while remaining completely detached from it all. In fact, a person in this subtype finds comfort in suffering and expressing it to others. This tends to generate attention, support and sometimes admiration from others.

They often feel inadequate about social situations and easily become envious of the social status of other people or when they meet those who seem to have already found a place where they "belong." A sense of belonging really drives them and they strive to establish an acceptable social role where they can be heavenly. Their biggest issue is being able to overcome the social shame they often experience, and there's always a hidden inner conflict going on because they constantly doubt themselves and struggle with feelings of inferiority. A person in this subtype will notice a tendency to blame others, compare himself with others, and constantly struggle with deep shame and envy.

Sexual Instinct:

The basic character drive will be competition.

If the previous subtype can be called shameful, then this personality variation can be called' shameless.'

This subtype is very loud and vocal about ha. With a lot of vigour, they express their emotions and desires. It's what I call the queen or king of the classic drama. They are highly demanding and highly competitive. Because they believe in evaluating themselves on the basis of how they match other people, competition is a major motivation for this subtype, and they will do anything to beat the competition.

Unfortunately, this competitiveness comes from a place of deep-seated insecurity and inadequacy feelings. For this subtype, personal blocks and issues are always resurfacing as their sense of value and value is directly linked to beating those they consider strong and powerful.

5. The Observer also called the Investigator.

Self-preservation Instinct:

The basic character drive here will be projected in the form of The Castle.

This variation in personality is driven by the need to be very protective of the place they call home. Their personal space and privacy are far beyond limits, and they have no difficulty in setting clear boundaries for all. They enjoy living a comfortable and relatively lonely life with a few close friends.

A person in this subtype would prefer to sit back and watch social life rather than participate actively in it. They are very guarded and independent in choosing to cut off intimacy so as not to lower their guard and lose that sense of privacy and security.

Having a safe haven where they can retreat and take refuge from the world is essential for this subtype. And because they also like seclusion, having enough supplies is always a concern for them, which often leads to a minimalist lifestyle being hoarded and lived.

However, some subtypes go to the other extreme and choose to make their' castle' wherever they are and end up traveling forever or moving from place to place. They tend to be introverts, but not all, and prefer not to reveal much of their inner world.

Social Instinct:

The basic character drive here will be projected in the form of symbols.

This variation of personality type is brilliant and hungry for more knowledge. Their main focus is on searching for meaning and answers to the most important life issues. They take little to no pleasure in dealing with trivia every day. Their hunger for mastery and understanding of sacred symbols and language leads them down paths that are rarely traversed by ordinary human beings.

This subtype loves to connect and engage with other brilliant minds and experts who share their ideas and hunger for higher knowledge and knowledge. Unfortunately, they often get too stuck in too much critical thinking, analysis and interpretation that causes a snag in their ability to participate actively with others.

A person in this subtype tends to be very private, reclusive and quiet, unwilling to share their personal space or inner resources, but at the same time, when triggered to talk about a topic they're passionate about, they'll be the same. It's almost as if they can go from being completely introverted to being energetically extroverted by pushing a button.

Sexual Instinct:

The basic character drive here is projected in the form of The Confidant.

This type five variation is the most person-related and connected. They love keeping things confidential too, but with this slight change. A subtype five confidant in a private one-on - one relationship will open up and share intimate information about their inner world and frame of mind. But only to a selected few who undergo a series of loyalty tests for the first time.

This subtype possesses the cooler and analytical character traits and although still super secretive and reserved, once they find that "shared chemistry" with another they open up and enjoy the trust and connection that such a relationship allows.

The main challenge this subtype struggles with is the creativity of tension. The Doubter also called the loyalist.

Instinct for self-preservation:

The basic character drive here will be projected as warmth.

This type six variation is very affectionate and warm-hearted. But they are very pronounced in fear, anxiety, and insecurity. They try to overcome it by building strong relationships and bonds that will help them feel safe.

You will often find that an earlier childhood event may have created a lot of suppressed hurt that causes them to be very afraid of taking risks or making mistakes. As a result, this subtype will prefer to repress their negative emotions, particularly because they see it as a better and more cautious way to deal with such feelings, especially if they believe it could jeopardize the warmth of a relationship they really need.

A person in this subtype doesn't like feeling "left out" and is struggling to share their opinions openly. They prefers to stay within well-established boundaries and risk-taking is not easy.

Social Instinct:

The basic character drive here will be projected as A Sense of Duty.

This type six variation of personality is very focused and concerned about living up to one's own duty. To those who belong to this subtype, integrity, fairness, and responsibility matter a lot. They believe in standing up for "the little guy" and defending the weak.

This subtype is highly rational and dedicated to their work, choosing to follow the rules and procedures set in their environment. They tend to be more black and white, connect with social ideals and enjoy working towards a greater cause.

A person in this subtype is very concerned about knowing the rules and making sure that everyone understands their role too often creating clear agreements with colleagues and friends to avoid confusion or unnecessary squabbling. The big challenge is the fear of rejection often brewing underneath and the deep sense of responsibility carried by their own duty which can either become a calling or a burden to them depending on how they develop their personality.

Sexual Instinct:

The basic character drive here will be projected as The Warrior.

This particular variation of personality type has two styles. The first style is based on overcoming the undercurrent of fear through physical strength and bravery's willpower and feats. It can also be seen in gaining intellectual power.

By creating beauty in their environment, the second style is seen. Channelling their idealism and keen perceptiveness into creating beauty in the hopes that it will help them feel more in control and stable.

Both styles within this subtype indicate a bold assertiveness that often leads to bullying. A person in this subtype will undoubtedly experience a lot of self-doubt, fear, and instability and will often try to avoid it or overcome it by either running straight to it through a focus on strength or beauty. This need for security and power often clouds their ability to connect with their own emotions and leads to a lot of vulnerability struggle.

7. The Dreamer also called the Enthusiast.

Self-preservation Instinct:

The fundamental character drive here will be projected in the form of networking.

This variation of personality type loves to have good things in life and is surrounded by rich relationships, beauty, fun conversations and entertainment.

They love planning fun projects or events, preparing elaborate meals, dinin. Despite being more interested in family and friends, their energetic and enthusiastic approach to life and people makes them great in nurturing a "family" relationship that extends far beyond blood relatives. What motivates them is to ensure that everyone does well and has the best experience with them.

A person in this subtype is usually very good at getting what they want and justifying or defending what they want to do. The biggest challenge is the tendency to overdo things, become too self-interested or overindulge in some way with food, talk, shopping or stimulants.

Social Instinct:

The basic character drive here will be projected as Sacrifice.

This subtype tends to act against the common feature of insatiability shown by the other seven. They are generous and have a strong desire to make meaning in the world and make a difference. They are pleased to sacrifice their own needs in order to serve the needs of the group, family, organization or person they support. They have a utopian outlook on life, which usually serves them well.

However, an underlying current of dependence is experienced with this subtype because they need friends and other people or group-based projects to express themselves and feel they are doing something meaningful. They secretly hope to be recognized and appreciated for the sacrifices they make in all their self-sacrificing nature.

A person in this subtype is very generous, visionary in their thinking, focuses more on others, and is attracted to anything that seeks to fulfill a greater cause. Their primary challenge is the tendency to be highly judgmental of others and of themselves whenever they perceive a sense of selfishness appearing.

Sexual Instinct:

The basic character drive here will be projected as Fascination.

Here we find the classical dreamer and idealist. This variant of personality type sees the world by means of rose-colored filters. They's immediately attracted to new ideas, new people and potential adventure falling into a state of fascination immediately. But this suggestibility works both ways.

Not only is this subtype easily fascinated, but it fascinates others as well. Their charm can be very persuasive and irresistible, making such people great when it comes to sales and customer service.

A person in this subtype sees the good in everything and is always excited and optimistic. They're always connected to the stream of infinite possibilities.

The main challenge is to deal with things They sees as dull, dreary, boring and predictable. Conditions, individuals and even a dull world are completely unacceptable and become a source of frustration.

8. The Challenger also called the Leader.

Self-preservation Instinct:

The basic drive of character here will be projected as Survival.

This variation of personality will be more driven and focused on survival and protecting those under their care. More interested in ensuring success and security in physical and materials. These subtype eights are aggressive and excessive in their tendencies.

A typical mind attitude is "win or die fighting." Usually, this subtype is seen as a very powerful, productive and direct personality that never supports situations simply because things get tough. They are also very fiercely protecting their family and friends and are often perceived as the strong pillar that holds things together.

A person in this subtype is confident, secure, powerful, direct and will usually assume the role of guardian, father or mother. They're very concerned about protecting themselves, their surroundings, and those under their care. Survival is a major concern at all times.

Social Instinct:

The basic character drive here will be projected as a camaraderie.

This personality variation of eight still has the same type eight aggression and excessiveness, but it can be channelled differently. A sense of injustice and powerlessness is active among the individuals who fall into this subtype, which they try to resolve by forming groups or alliances to which they are very dedicated.

They focus more on social causes and prefer to be the group or alliance leader, serving the people for a higher mission. Unfairness, injustice or abuse of power triggers their sensitivities and they feel the need to protect against such things those under their influence. They prefer to support others rather than assert their own personal needs.

A person in this subtype will usually choose to mediate their anger by harnessing that energy to serve the needs of the members of the community they serve. They will also want to be the "shield" loyally protecting his or her tribe from unjust authority or any other type of danger.

Sexual instinct:

The fundamental character drive here will be projected as possessiveness.

This type eight variation demands control over others and loves to possess whatever they desire. They like being rebellious and have no fear of breaking the rules. Impulsive rules for this subtype, and very intense people are usually always ready to disrupt things and bring about change. They will never shy away from challenging the status quo and will need to drive change, gain power and influence over others.

When it comes to intimacy, the eight aggressions and possessively are still very pronounced, often wanting to dominate the partner entirely.

A person in this subtype will have the same aggressive and excessive qualities as all types eight, but with one distinct qualities. They're going to tend to take it a little too far.

There's a hunger for possession that can sometimes be good if it's aimed at serving a worthy cause. But if it's directed to something detrimental for them and others, it can also be dangerous. Sometimes this subtype of personality may be willing to let go and surrender if They feels a strong enough desire from a partner able to fully meet their needs.

9. The Peacemaker also called the Diplomat.

Self-preservation Instinct:

The basic character drive here will be projected as a Strong Appetite.

This personality variation is somewhat similar to an eight subtype in that they are very self-focused and concerned about meeting physical needs.

Material safety and the provision of daily comfort is very important. Those who fall into this subtype have a great appetite for food and possessing things.

A person is often a collector in this subtype. Very focused on meeting their personal needs and providing comfort to the material. They loves time alone and can become very irritable when someone threatens their sense of equilibrium or disrupts the daily rhythms that support their instinctual life. Material abundance is often more important than personal or spiritual growth.

Social Instinct:

The basic drive will be projected as a Powerful Need for Participation.

This variation in personality of the nine is the most friendly, selfless and warm type. Those who are in this subtype are usually strong, reliable, always in harmony with others and do a great job blending in with their friends ' agenda or the different social groups they become part of.

This subtype, often showing excellent leadership skills and selfless contribution, will position itself as the mediator or facilitator that comes naturally to them. Their instinctual motive is to be part of a wider group or the community benefactor. They don't like to burden others with their personal struggles so they usually maintain a happy attitude and focus on other people's needs and roles.

A person in this subtype is more interested in just feeling like they're participating in something meaningful. They's working hard to make those they love happy and willing to make whatever sacrifices are necessary to meet the needs of those under their care.

They are affectionate and friendly to do their utmost to be a reliable, concrete pillar for those in their care, even if it means neglecting their own pain and struggles.

Sexual Instinct:

The fundamental character drives here wil Union with others is their instinctual motive, and that can be either sexual or spiritual with another person, nature, or lifeitself.

This deep longing may sometimes be chaotic, or it may be the gateway to a transcendental experience. When partnered with others, they tend to feel more comfortable and secure and usually can not stand alone. As a result, there may be a tendency to go along with other people's demands and exclude their personal preferences.

A person in this subtype is usually very warm and affectionate with a deep urge for fusion. Their most important challenge is to make this practical in day-to-day living and keeping personal boundaries as well as focusing on oneself.

How to know your Subtype:

Before moving on to the next section, here are a few tips on how to recognize your subtype. This could be easy for some people. You could take the Enneagram test in a matter of minutes and figure out your center and subtypes. I'm happy if that's you. You're fine to go. Simply apply everything you've learned as you move forward in life.

However, if you're not that lucky and still feel lost, confused or even unable to figure out your subtype instantly, I've covered you. You're not on your own. This is something that is happening to many people. It requires more study and exploration over time, so let the process evolve naturally.

I think we all identify with all three instinctual drives to some extent. So if you find that's just knowing that there's nothing wrong with you. After all, in each of us, they all exist.

But what is the most important thing for you in general? This is the clarity you need.

The subtypes of the Enneagram are not meant to be an accurate science. Rather, they are meant to evoke a specific theme and make you aware of the various seasons in your life and the different motives that influence your choices. The Enneagram personality tool is a dynamic growth-oriented system and is meant to be a personal inventory that aims to identify your basic fears motivations and strengths so that through a specific trajectory you can facilitate your personal growth.

If you can start by confidently identifying your primary type and the main intelligence center (one of the triads), then you will be able to discover. As you determine what to identify with, avoid becoming too rigid about this.

Look at the diagram I share below. A visual representation of your subtypes should be given to you. You may choose to start first by identifying with the most attractive instinct center. For example: If you feel genuinely driven by social instinct and the need to belong or fight for a higher cause within a group, then you can focus on the-social instinct-and match your Enneagram type to the corresponding subtype.

Self Preservation Instinct	Social Instinct	Sexual Instinct
The need to preserve our body and its life force. Keeping away from threats. This includes our basic human needs of food, shelter, clothing, warmth and family relations.	The need to get along with others and form secure social bonds. It's about creating a sense of belonging around you.	The universal need to procreate and continue the human race generation after generation. It governs our sexuality, intimacy and the close friendships that we treasure as well as our legacy.
Type 1: The Perfectionist /Reformer	**Type 1: The Perfectionist /Reformer**	**Type 1: The Perfectionist /Reformer**
•Anxiety	•Non-adaptability	•Zealousness or Jealousy
Type 2: The Giver/Helper	**Type 2: The Giver/Helper**	**Type 2: The Giver/Helper**
•Privilege	•Ambition	•Seduction or Aggression
Type 3: The Achiever/Performer	**Type 3: The Achiever/Performer**	**Type 3: The Achiever/Performer**
•Security	•Prestige	•Charisma
Type 4: The Romantic/Individualist	**Type 4: The Romantic/Individualist**	**Type 4: The Romantic/Individualist**
•Fearlessness	•Shame	•Competition
Type 5: The Observer/Investigator	**Type 5: The Observer/Investigator**	**Type 5: The Observer/Investigator**
•Castle	•Symbols	•Confidant
Type 6: The Loyalist/Doubter	**Type 6: The Loyalist/Doubter**	**Type 6: The Loyalist/Doubter**
•Warmth	•Duty	•Warrior
Type 7: The Enthusiast/Dreamer	**Type 7: The Enthusiast/Dreamer**	**Type 7: The Enthusiast/Dreamer**
•Networking	•Sacrifice	•Fascination
Type 8: The Challenger/Leader	**Type 8: The Challenger/Leader**	**Type 8: The Challenger/Leader**
•Survival	•Camaraderie	•Possessiveness
Type 9: The Peacemaker/Diplomat	**Type 9: The Peacemaker/Diplomat**	**Type 9: The Peacemaker/Diplomat**
•Strong Appetite	•Participation	•Fusion

If that doesn't seem to yield clear results, try a different approach. Within the subtypes that most resonate with you, you may choose to write down all the nine sets. You'll probably feel more attracted to one of the sets of nine terms than the other two. The one that attracts you most should be the instinctual title that best describes your long-run habits, concerns, and anxieties.

My friend Joanna was at first struggling to identify her subtype. She thought she was a type four Enneagram personality with her dominant subtype being the instinct of self-preservation. Her husband was not in agreement. This created some doubt in her, and before she finally felt comfortable with her chosen Enneagram type and subtype, it took a lot of studies and deep reflection. Maybe at first you'll need to do the same. Keep going and let the drawings below guide you into your truth.

Section IV:

Using The Enneagram To Enrich Your Life

Chapter 08: Integrating an ancient tool into a modern living

There's no denying that the model of the Enneagram is as simple as it is profoundly complex.

The layers on the Enneagram system as shown in the previous chapter are then dissected. Fortunately for you, it won't take you a decade.

In fact, all you need to get started on your self-discovery is to take a test to learn your type in the nine-point system and figure out your subtype, so you can be well on your way to profound revelations about your behaviour, your strengths and how to grow.

The more you understand why you're doing what you're doing, the easier it's going to be for you. At the very least, you'll have a fresh new lens to interact with and understand those you meet in your everyday life. That is the power of the Enneagram.

This system, passed on for generations from ancient times to modern times, can become a handy tool for your personal growth, conflict resolution, and even development of characters.

Are there areas in your life that you have been struggling with?

Do you have painful relationships because you just don't seem to be able to make them work the way you think they should work? Are there people in your workplace or you can't see eye to eye at home, yet you know that you just have to find a way to get along because of the commitments that you have made?

Is it your body that just doesn't seem to listen or respond positively to anything you're trying to do?

All these issues can be improved with the use of this tool.

Chapter 09: Accelerating your personal growth and self-expression

Personal growth and self-expression are as essential as breathing for us as human beings.

All these issues can be improved with the use of this tool. The desire for self-expression arises naturally once we secure the basic needs that help us to feel safe and comfortable. It's meant to be part of our evolution and self-realization.

Self-expression doesn't necessarily mean that art is produced, written, performed, or any of that. It may necessarily include that for some people, but at its core, it's about communicating your truth and using body language, your work and actions, and how you interact and engage in your world with others. This also includes how you dress, how you drive your car, how you decorate your home, etc.

The main challenge with personal growth and self-expression comes when there feels like there's a block or a lack of inspiration and creativity to get through something you want to portray to someone else in some way.

If you've ever been in a situation where you really wanted to express something that was weighing on your heart, but for whatever reason you've not been able to get this emotion out.

This is a common problem when we do not yet understand the motives, instincts and behaviours that affect our personalities. We may have an idea of what we want to communicate, but we are short on execution or full demonstration.

The other day I was watching a baking show, and one of the contestants competing to win $10,000 started crying when her cake looked like nothing she had imagined in her mind. Even the judges had a hard time scoring her because they could see her anguish and the fact that she couldn't manifest whatever creative idea she had at the start of the competition.

The reason why personality tool Enneagram works so well to improve people's lives is because it helps them better understand their strengths, hang-ups, instinctual drives and warning signs to watch. This tool also highlights the underlying fears that often guide our behaviour.

Don Richard Riso and Russ Hudson reveal the nine core fears that everyone needs to be aware of in "The Wisdom of The Enneagram."

Type One: Fear of being evil or corrupt.

This type of personality strives to be morally upright and virtuous in the face of external corruption. They tend to be perfectionist, sweating even minute details at all times. And their underlying fear is corruption. So the drive for meticulousness and virtual action is driven by the need to prove that fear is wrong. Motivated by their own sense of integrity, individuals who are type one personality will constantly strive to move away from corruption to virtue.

Type Two: fear of being unloved or unwanted by others

This type of personality strives to be loved and desired by those around them. They give, nurture and invest a lot of their time, effort and resources to cultivate relationships in order to overcome the inherent fear of not being lovable. The giving and helping that comes from people in the type two personality comes from a place where they prove that they deserve to be cared for and loved by others because they give it too much. They will constantly strive to move away from worthlessness and towards relationships that foster mutual love and caregiving.

Type Three: fear of being worthless and unfulfilled

This type of personality aims to achieve success and status quo as the right measure of their own worth. The underlying fear here is a sense of worthlessness inherent in it. This type feels that they are not desirable apart from their accomplishments and must therefore accomplish as much as possible to be desired and accepted by others. They will strive to move continuously from worthlessness to impressive achievements that can earn great admiration and respect.

Type Four: fear of lacking a unique, special and significant identity.

With this type of personality comes the need to prove to others their uniqueness and individuality. The underlying fear in personality type four is that They would be unworthy and unlovable if they were "ordinary" or "average." As such, they seek to create a unique identity to prove their meaning in the world.

Those who are a personality type four are constantly moving from normal to expressions of individuality and intensity. They are afraid to be helpless, overwhelmed and unable to deal with the world around them. As a result, they try to learn as much as they can and master as much as they can to feel safe, skilled and able to handle the world. Those in this type of personality are constantly striving to move away from ignorance and ambiguity towards knowledge and understanding.

Type Six: Fear of being without support or guidance.

This type six personality is striving to find guidance and support from those around them. Their underlying fear is that they themselves are unable to survive. As such, they always seek as much other people's support and direction as possible. Those who fall into this type of personality are constantly striving to move away from isolation and towards other people's structure, security, and guidance.

Type Seven: Fear of deprivation and pain

This type seven personality strives to achieve their wildest desires and find satisfaction. Their underlying concern is that their needs and desires will not be met by others. Rather, they feel they have to go and pursue on their own what they want. Those in this type of personality strive to move away from pain, sadness, and helplessness toward independence, happiness, and fulfilment.

Type 8: fear of being harmed or controlled by others

This type of personality strives to be independent, powerful, influential, and self-directed. Their underlying concern is to be betrayed, controlled, or otherwise violated. This type of personality can not be controlled or at the mercy of others. Only when they are in control of their circumstances do they feel safe and fine. Those who fall into this type of personality are constantly moving away from outside limitations to self-sufficiency and power.

Type Nine: fear of loss and separation from others.

This type of personality strives to maintain harmony and peace both internally and externally. Their underlying fear is that they will be separated from others and disconnected. They're afraid the world around them will go out of sync. As such, they will do all they can to live in harmony with other people and the world around them because this creates a sense of security and connectivity. Those in this type of personality usually strive to move away from conflict and pain and toward stability, peace, and harmony.

By understanding your primary type of Enneagram, your basic fears, and your subtype, your natural gifts are fully appreciated, and limitations are not so mysterious.

It becomes easier to find satisfaction in your work and relationships. You'll better equipped to handle situations, hostile environments, and impulsive behaviours. For instance, if you have a deep longing for others to feel positively about you, you might have problems knowing when to say "no" to something because you're predisposed to wanted to please people. So maybe if you're asked to do double shifts at work, you might say, "yes," even if it hurts you. In such a situation, learning to say "no" would be the healthier, more satisfying answer, yet you would only have this awareness of yourself if you really understood more about your personality type.

Some people can quickly spot their primary and subtype personalities while it takes time, study and constant self-reflection for others. I don't know how long it's going to take you, but I encourage you to start because the sooner you do, the faster you're going to be able to create a healthier, more balanced life. Before moving on to the impact and benefit of using this tool and the insights gained to improve your relationships, I invite you to take the Enneagram test and discover your primary type as well as your wings, center and subtype.

Chapter 10: Enneagram Test

Let's take a quick look at the main personality types before you jump into our interactive online test:

Type 1: Reformer

If this is you, then you're not once to hesitate. You're purpose driven, set high standards for yourself, and are very self-controlled.

Type Two: Helper

If this is your primary type, then you're driven by the need for others to be loved and cared for. You're generous, compassionate, humble, and uplifting. There's a deep desire to feel loved and accepted, and sometimes the gift can be made in an effort to secure that state of love.

Type Three: Attain

If this is your primary type, then you're more focused on being the best. You want others to perceive you as being successful. You're usually very assertive, winning is all, and it matters a lot to your personal image.

Type Four: Romantic

If this is your primary type, then you have an impeccable eye for beauty in everything you do. You're more attuned to your and others ' emotions and can be quite dramatic at times. You're a romantic at heart, and a sanctuary to be treasured is your inner fantasy world.

Type Five: Observer

If this is your primary type, concentrate on knowledge and gain more knowledge. With a deep hunger for new ideas and greater understanding, you're highly intellectual. You can articulate new paradigms in a visionary way, and although you prefer isolation, when you're invited to speak on a topic, you can be very welcoming and engaged.

Type six: Loyalist

If this is your core personality type, then you're full of courage. You're self-confident and trustworthy. You often struggle with self-doubt and doubt others, which can create a rollercoaster of emotions for you, but you're very committed and decisive when you're not in doubt.

Type 7: Enthusiast

If this is your primary type, then fun and spontaneity is your thing. Being around you is fun, playful and pleasant. You have a very positive outlook and savour the world's wealth. However, you tend to get distracted easily, and you always seem to be moving to the next exciting adventure, but if you're not scattered around or distracted, you have the potential for tremendous accomplishments.

Type 8: Challenger

If this is your primary type, then you're intense! You like to be with others directly. You're concerned about productivity, high energy and excellence in your work. You're self-determined, generous, and you have a big heart. Others generally perceive you as very powerful, which can sometimes make you seem somewhat intimidating and controlling, especially when you try to gain control and influence over others.

Type nine: Peacemaker

Peace and harmony are your primary driver if you fall into a type nine personality. You're authentic, unpretentious, and patient, you get along with everybody, you love serving others, and you put your needs first. At your best, you can recognize, encourage and help bring out the best in others.

Take the test now and once you have your results to go back to section II to read a more in-depth description of your type, then jump into section III to find out what kind of layered cake you have.

To access the test, simply copy and paste the following link into your browser:

https://bit.ly/2xEWljl

Remember what we said about the subtypes being like layers of a cake that we all have?

It means that you already have all three basic instincts, but one is going to be more dominant. By discovering how your cake is layered, you will begin to be more awake in your daily choices, and some of your impulses, reactions, and experiences will make more sense.

You're a type of personality combined with your wings and center as well as your layered basic instincts now give you a detailed understanding of what makes you tick. And what a release that becomes as you step into improving your relationships with others.

Chapter 11: Cultivating Healthy Loving Relationships

Cultivating healthy, nourishing relationships is vital to us all. But we know how tough it can be with constant demands, especially in our modern society. That's why choosing your relationships wisely is even more critical than ever before.

The people you associate with and invest your energy both personally and professionally impact your well-being and success directly. That's why I encourage you to get better with the right people around you. But who is the right person?

In particular, when introducing Enneagram type combinations, a critical point to remember here is that no paring is particularly blessed or doomed to work out. The mistake so many people make is to avoid or undervalue all the other types once they learn about these Enneagram combinations. Focusing on a particular combination doesn't guarantee that you will be happy, nourished and in love.

What you want to achieve is another goal. You want to make sure the healthy versions of your types are displayed by both you and the person concerned. As long as two of you (regardless of type) are healthy, it will be amazing to experience together.

This is not always the norm, unfortunately. That's where it comes to play with self-discovery and further education. The better you're informed about the type, health level and tendencies of the other person, the greater your insight into the relationship. This is such a great tool to help you deepen your relationships as it will make you both aware of your behaviours. Once you shed light on your underlying fears, motives and natural tendencies as well as your gifts, you will have a choice as to how to respond to relationships in your life.

Regardless of your current needs for relationships, whether it's building healthy professional relationships with customers or cultivating a passionate, intimate relationship with your significant other. It will help you to love more in the present and to have a more grounded experience in your true nature. Finally, when you act out of fear and when you act out of your own truth, you will be able to recognize. It will also enable you to discern the desires of your true self and those that are superficial.

It becomes easy to love and live in harmony with others once you have this level of clarity and self-awareness. Instead of reacting when things don't go the way you want in a relationship, you'll feel empowered to react with love, support, encourage, and bring out the best in others. You'll also become a better communicator, more importantly. And we all know how important communication is in a healthy relationship.

One of my best friends has recently experienced the power to use this Enneagram tool to help both her self-discovery and her fiancé.

There's no doubt in her mind how much Tom loves her. He's the most generous, warm, appreciative, careful, playful, and nurturing man she's ever met. They make the perfect couple because their personality seems to be complimented by him. She says, "I feel so loved and special when I'm with him. There's no one else I'd like to marry, but at times he can be somewhat controlling, needy and insincere, and it really created friction between us."

That was before I suggested that both of them study the Enneagram. She had already taken the test, so it wasn't too far-fetched an idea, but before Tom agreed it took a little bit of convincing. She told me her relationship had completely transformed in less than a month. She's found new ways to show her love and feels more compassion when some of her weaknesses appear.

They have increased their level of intimacy and communication. Above all, their behaviors are less like a mysterious enemy trying to sabotage one another's love. I can only assume that their self-discoveries will enrich their future marriage even more.

Although I will choose to focus more on personal and intimate relationships, the same concept can be applied to any relationship with which you wish to work.

Returning the magic of passionate love:

There's nothing more exciting than finding someone who "gets you." When you have discovered your type of Enneagram and use it to improve as well as enhance who you really are, it will change how you approach relationships forever.

This is not a reading of the horoscope, but a tool to use to determine the best type of people that will complement and enhance your whole life. I'm not saying it's an exact science, but when you learn about the personality types of your loved ones, you'll be amazed at how harmonious your relationships will be. The tendencies that usually hold you back from having healthy relationships with yourself and others won't be a mystery anymore. After all, the happier you become, the easier it will be to nurture healthy relationships.

Suggested combination types from the Enneagram Institute:

There are some insights into relationships for each type that could be a great starting point if you're looking for new loving relationships to manifest:

Type 1: The Perfectionist or Reformer

Best type combinations: 1 2 3 4 5 6 7 8 9

Type 2: The Giver or Helper

Best type combinations: 1 2 3 4 5 6 7 8 9

Type 3: The Achiever or Performer

Best type combinations: 1 2 3 4 5 6 7 8 9

Type 4: The Romantic or Individualist

Best type combinations: 1 2 3 4 5 6 7 8 9

Type 5: The Observer or Investigator

Best type combinations: 1 2 3 4 5 6 7 8 9

Type 6: The Loyalist or Doubter

Best type combinations: 1 2 3 4 5 6 7 8 9

Type 7: The Enthusiast or Dreamer

Best type combinations: 1 2 3 4 5 6 7 8 9

Type 8: The Challenger or Leader

Best type combinations: 1 2 3 4 5 6 7 8 9

Type 9: The Peacemaker or Diplomat

Best type combinations: 1 2 3 4 5 6 7 8 9

I know it's hard to hear, but if you kick your heels back and relax once in a while, the world won't crumble. Release the need for constant monitoring of each outcome. It's also great to share your core values and motivations openly with your loved ones. Let them know how much you care and invite them into that vision to improve the world. Those who "get you" will be more than just encouraging your tendencies and supporting them.

Type Two: The Giver

Having discovered that you're warm, empathetic and motivated by the need to be loved and needed, this is your suggestion for a relationship.

Fight the urge to always jump in and fix the problems of other people, even if you're great at it. Learn to be there without getting too absorbed in their world for your significant other and often step out of the box to get in touch with your feelings. Ask yourself, "How am I doing?"

Type Three: The Achiever

Discovering that you're motivated by success, winning big, and being wired for high performance and productivity, here is your suggestion for a relationship.

You have a lot to offer, not just material success and social status. Connect to the "more" you have. You're not always bound by someone's appreciation and value to your accomplishments. Learn how to make authentic connections and do not shy away from deep diving under the prestige and material success you have.

Type Four: The Romantic

Having discovered that you're a natural romantic with an eye for beauty and that you're more creative and expressive than most, here is your suggestion for a relationship.

Learn to take control of your emotions or they will control you and create constant problems. Without consuming you, you can become more aware of your emotions. Since you know, there's a tendency to be a queen or king of drama and that you're particularly sensitive when you feel misunderstood, communicate this to your loved one and help them know this side of you so that when it happens they too can respond accordingly. Use your power of perception to put yourself in the shoes of the one you love so that you can see things from their side of the table, then you will always know the right thing to do in any given situation.

Type Five: The Observer

Having discovered that you're the private, analytical type motivated by a hunger to gain more knowledge, here is your suggestion for a relationship. Just do it! Don't worry about being "pulled in" close by someone else where chemistry aligns. Your feelings are not too much to be dealt with by someone else, and you have what it takes to be good at this. Learn to reconnect more with your heart so that you can know when it's time to make the shift from head to heart.

Type Six: The Loyalist

Having discovered that you're the practical, committed, but always anxious type, here's your suggestion for your relationship.

Not everyone has a "hidden agenda." I know it's hard to hear and you're having a hard time being optimistic, but it's not going to make you feel optimistic. Your ability to be a great and loyal friend, always reliable and trustworthy, is a power that should not be underestimated in our modern world in particular. Learn how to use this power to build a robust and reliable bond with a significant other.

Type 7: The Enthusiast

With the new discovery of your type as fun, spontaneous and motivated by pleasure searching for experiences that stimulate you, here's your relationship advice.

Your positive, fun-loving attitude is contagious and will always attract great people to you, but you have to do it. Find the courage to face what might drive you to activities that are restless and shallow. It's not such a bad thing you know to be committed to the right person? You have so much greatness and wisdom to offer that you start to work on being more focused on body and mind.

Type 8: The Challenger

There's no doubt about it, you're fierce and intense. You're powerful, full of energy, strong and motivated by a need to control the underdogs and protect them. Here's a relationship tip that can help you cultivate amazing connections.

Vulnerability is not a bad thing in their eyes, especially with the one you love. Be all right to express any emotions that come up for you. The real you can be handled by people who love you. The real power you possess is the ability to show strength and tenderness when the situation demands it. Don't hold back or fight those rare moments as they become your most magical with the one you love.

Type Nine: The Peacemaker

Having discovered that you're the laid-back, harmonious guy who always gets along with everybody here is a piece of advice for you.

Yes, you're a peacemaker, but you don't always have to "settle" for something if you don't really want it. And being the wonderful mediator you're, even if they differ, it can be easier to express your needs and desires to someone else. Although it makes you uncomfortable, you have permission to voice a contrasting opinion to your significant other. The one who really loves you will appreciate your knowledge of the frame of mind and perspective of things even more. So go on, tell your truth!

Chapter 12: Mapping your most joyful and fulfilling path

As we said at the beginning of our journey in self-discovery and understanding of the Enneagram, this typing system is based on an ancient practice developed over the years to help us apply it better.

The modern Enneagram as we know it's divided into a nine-point system and subdivided into three triads or centres. The triads represent the head, the heart, and the gut, alternatively referred to as the center of thought, the center of feeling, and the center of instincts, which form the essential components of the human psyche.

While there are so many personality-typing systems available today, the Enneagram stands out from the crowd and for this particular reason maintains its global merit. Not only does it plunge deeper into variations that you will experience even within your dominant type, it also adds a unique aspect to things.

Namely:

You're given the direction of integration, which explains how your type is likely to behave on a health and growth pathway. And you're also given the direction of disintegration, which describes how your type is likely to act under pressure and stress.

This means that your self-discovery goes much deeper than the usual personality typing systems because it gives you the power to introspect and make new conscious choices in any area of your life, including relationships. For anyone interested in taking their personal growth and self-awareness to the next level, it's a vital tool.

The Enneagram is a tool designed to help you observe your personality (ego) and how it works closer. Being aware of who you really are, the basic instincts that drive your behavior and the quality of character that you can build to create either a healthy progressive path in life or a disintegrative path is the beginning of your self-discovery.

Depending on your core personality type, there are some passions to become vigilant and work towards transformation at a fundamental level. The more you reflect on your behaviors and motives, the easier it will be to turn them into healthy virtues because, as you recall at the beginning of the book, we affirmed that each of us is pure and good in essence.

Here is a quick recap of the passions or behaviors that may unconsciously govern your life, plus how to transform them into healthy virtues. By taking the online test to which we provided the link in a previous chapter, the best way to figure out your type is. By answering all the questions honestly, your top score will show you what type of personality you are. Bear in mind, you might have multiple high scores because, as we said, the Enneagram is a complex, interconnected system just as a human being is complex and therefore can not be rigidly restricted to just one strict type.

Alternatively, you could go back to the earlier chapters and read through all the detailed descriptions of all personality types and try to decide which one is yours. If you feel that you know yourself well enough to identify your type instantly, then you can continue to study and understand your chosen type and all the additional information that we have shared in this book.

How the Enneagram can help you grow and manifest a joy-filled life.

The Enneagram is like a roadmap that empowers your self-observation capability and shows you how to reach higher levels of consciousness. The more you develop a clear vision of the healthiest and best version you can be, the more your life will be joyful and prosperous. It can be as simple as you want it to be, or as complex. Beginning with the basics is recommended. This book covers all the basics and some in-depth understanding of the system's intricacies. That doesn't mean that our studies end there, though. You can still dive deeper into your self-determined core personality type, wings and subtype by venturing into what is referred to as developmental levels.

In 1977, Don Riso discovered and began developing what is now known as the nine developmental levels which are the internal structures that make up the personality type itself. In other words, what Don Riso teaches is that you have an internal structure that is the core of your personality. There are layers within these internal structures and a certain behavioral demonstration of your personality type will be pronounced depending on your level. The range extends from healthy, average, and down to lower, unhealthy levels.

Don Riso and Russ Hudson further enhanced this discovery in the 1990s. They are the only Enneagram teachers in their Enneagram teachings to include this internal structure. The book recommended in chapter nine "The Enneagram's Wisdom" can also help you better understand what these teachers mean by levels of development plus how to rise higher in your development.

They have developed these nine levels of development to provide a "skeletal" structure of each type that can be very useful for therapists, counselors and other medical professions working with a client. By learning more about the nine levels of development within their personality type and where they are at a given time along that continuum, you can understand whether the person works within the healthy, average or unhealthy range and support them accordingly. Don Riso has other books available online, but I specifically encourage you to check out the The Wisdom of The Enneagram if you feel ready to dive into more details about your core personality. With the information shared in this book alone, you can quickly improve your work, health relationships and overall lifestyle. So if you don't want to be an expert on this, don't worry. You already have all the knowledge you need to enhance your self-reflection and awareness ability. Naturally, the rest will unfold as you continue to work on understanding yourself and improving the areas of weakness that come to your conscious awareness.

Now that you have made the first few steps forward, there's no return. You can never be the same again for your work, relationships and how you perceive yourself. You will have a better chance of controlling yourself in whatever environment or situation you end up in if you have done the inner work. Planning for your future goals will also have more confidence. Having this inner and outer equilibrium is what you need in our modern world to thrive as your true self. Now that you're better at understanding and getting the tool out and cultivating the quality of life you've always wanted!

Made in the USA
Las Vegas, NV
11 December 2021

37154182R00069